Yoga For Beginners:

Your Beginners Guide to Yoga for Weight Loss, Stress Relief and Inner Peace

SID AKULA

ISBN: **1511705183**
ISBN-13: **978-1511705189**

CONTENTS

INTRODUCTION

"To liberate the potential of your mind, body, and soul, you must first expand your imagination. You see, things are always created twice: first in the workshop of the mind and then, and only then, in reality." -Robin Sharma, *The Monk Who Sold His Ferrari*

Yoga is so much more than an exercise or a fitness routine. It is a change in your lifestyle that will make you feel better: mind, body, and soul. Yoga is the science of "right" living, and it is a complete lifestyle change that will transform everything from your body to you mind to your interactions with other people. It works on and advances all characteristics of the person: the physical, the mental, the emotional, the psychic and the spiritual. When broken down, the word yoga means "unity" or "oneness" and is derived from the Sanskrit word "yuj" which roughly means "to join."

There are too many misconceptions clouding the benefits science of yoga. For far too long, people have viewed it as a "weak" exercise or something for suburban mothers, hippies, or celebrities. People also think that it is some kind of gymnastics or stretching routine, a type physical or mental debauchery through which miraculous feats can be performed while wearing stretch clothes and repeating phrases. While some of that can be true some of the time, everyone's experience with yoga is different. For some who practice yoga, it is an extremely dangerous practice in which they can pull muscles, pop joints, or pass out. Few people think of yoga as the kind of mental and physical acrobatics that is compatible only with a Hindu mind and found only in those who practice for quite a long time.

The human mind has been proven to have certain weaknesses which are universal. Many define them as:

- Avidya-wrong notions of the external world
- Asmita-wrong notions of oneself
- Raga-longing and attachment for sensory objects and affections
- Dweshad-like and hatred for objects and persons
- Abinivesha-the love of life

These are the five defects of the human mind that must be removed or categorized. Yoga is the constant meditation and introspection that seeks to eradicate these mental flaws.

In this book, I have organized some background information on understanding yoga better, determine if it is for you, explain the benefits and give you the skills you need to be completely comfortable starting out.

This journey is yours and yours alone – but we can help you get there.

Let's get started…

WHY YOGA?

"Your life is a sacred journey. It is about change, growth, discovery, movement, transformation, continuously expanding your vision of what is possible, stretching your soul, learning to see clearly and deeply, listening to your intuition, taking courageous challenges at every step along the way. You are on the path... exactly where you are meant to be right now... And from here, you can only go forward, shaping your life story into a magnificent tale of triumph, of healing, of courage, of beauty, of wisdom, of power, of dignity, and of love." -Caroline Adams

There are some people who doubt yoga and think that it really has no health benefits. In truth, the number of benefits is immeasurable because it depends on the individual person, the type of yoga practiced, and the amount of effort put into the program. These are just some of the most popular benefits though there are many others. Practice yoga and see your own benefits, as they will be sure to surprise you, delight you, and fill you with glee.

Stress Relief

Yoga reduces the physical effects of stress on the body and on the mind through simplifying and pushing negative energy away. By encouraging relaxation and meditation, yoga helps to lower the levels of what actually causes stress, the hormone cortisol. Related benefits of lowering stress levels include lowering blood pressure and overall heart rate, improving digestion and boosting the immune system, as well as easing the overall symptoms of detrimental conditions such as anxiety, depression, bipolar disorder, fatigue, asthma, diabetes, and insomnia.

Pain Relief

Yoga can also ease pain for some people. Studies have demonstrated that people who are practicing yoga asanas (postures), meditation, a combination of the two, or many other types of yoga for an extended period of time had reduced pain for those with conditions such as cancer, multiple sclerosis, auto-immune diseases, and hypertension as well as things like arthritis, back and neck pain, and other chronic conditions. Some specialists even suggest that perhaps emotional pain from daily events (like stress) can be eased through the practice of yoga.

Enhanced Breathing Techniques

Yoga teaches people to take slower, deeper breaths from deeper within the diaphragm – similar to those taken while singing or playing an instrument. This helps to improve the lung function, triggering the body's relaxation response and increasing the amount of oxygen available to the body. This leads to increased healing, better exercise, and overall health. Yoga has been shown to be good for people trying to quit smoking because it helps restore the lungs and remove the toxins.

Improve Flexibility

Yoga helps to improve a person's flexibility and mobility, increasing the range of movement possible while reducing the aches and pains felt with that motion and other motions. Many people can't even touch their toes during their first yoga class, but that will change quickly! Gradually, they will begin to use the correct muscles, including muscles that don't move or stretch with daily life. Over time, the ligaments, tendons, and muscles lengthen, increasing elasticity, making more poses possible as well as increasing the movement that is possible during the day. Yoga also helps to improve body alignment, causing the person to have better posture and helping to relieve back, neck, joint, and muscle problems. Many have also said that the improved flexibility has led to a better sex life.

Increased Strength

Yoga asanas (postures) uses every single muscle in the body, pushing it, at times, to the limit and helping to increase a person's strength from head to toe and fingertip to fingertip. The best part is that while these postures strengthen the body and build lean muscles, they also provide an additional benefit of helping to relieve muscular tension. This will make those long, lean muscles that are still defined, but don't bulge out in a way that isn't attractive to some.

Weight Management and Weight Loss

Yoga, even the less vigorous styles and practices, can aid a person's weight control efforts by reducing the cortisol levels within the body as well as by burning excess calories and reducing stress which encourages poor food choices. Yoga also encourages healthy eating habits and provides a heightened sense of well-being and self-esteem. A person practicing yoga is more likely to make a good food choice and is more likely to continue exercising – unlike people who start running on a treadmill or working out on an elliptical.

Improved Circulation

Yoga helps to improve blood circulation and, as a result of various poses in all practices, more efficiently moves oxygenated blood to the body's cells. This is why many athletes will practice yoga, as an increased blood flow will help muscles repair themselves and will lead to a body that can systematically combat the breakdown and mass loss.

Cardiovascular Training

Even gentle yoga practices that don't require sweating or heavy breathing can provide cardiovascular benefits to the participant by lowering the resting heart rate, increasing overall endurance, and improving oxygen uptake during exercise. This makes yoga a great choice for marathoners and even those with stress problems. It teaches coping methods that help increase focus.

Improved Focus and Consciousness

Yoga helps us to focus on what is truly important: the present, causing to become more aware of our space on earth and to help create mind and body health. It opens the door to improved concentration, coordination, reaction time, and memory. In this way, it is often great for young children with attention disorders as it calms then and gives them a point of focus.

Inner Peace

Perhaps one of the top reasons to practice yoga, the meditative aspects of yoga help many to reach a deeper, more divine, and more nourishing place in their lives. Many who begin to practice for other reasons, such as weight loss or health, have reported this to be a key reason that yoga has become an essential part of their daily lives and the reason they continue.

If you start trying yoga for one reason, chances are you will stay for another. Yoga has so many benefits that are small, but extremely helpful to creating a life that is wholesome and healthy. Yoga isn't just another thing to do at the gym, it is a way to change up your lifestyle and embrace your health without having to worry about passing out or getting your heart rate up too high.

Yoga is a gentle giant when it comes to your health.

YOGA STYLES

"I have been a seeker and I still am, but I stopped asking the books and the stars. I started listening to the teaching of my Soul." - Rumi

There are many different styles of yoga being taught and practiced today all over the world. Most communities will have at least a few styles of yoga. However, there isn't a studio near you that practices that particular type of yoga, there are resources online to help one practice at home. Although all of the styles are grounded in the same basic physical postures (called poses), each has a particular emphasis or goal. Here is just a quick guide on the most popular types of yoga worldwide that can help you decode the schedule at your gym, wade through those YouTube videos, and figure out which class is right for you, your body, and your goals.

Let's examine the different Schools of Yoga.

Anusara

Developed by an American yogi named John Friend in 1997, Anusara yoga is sort of like the younger brother to most of the yoga world. It is also the most popular type of yoga taught in the United States. Based on the belief that everyone on earth is filled with an intrinsic goodness, Anusara yoga's goal is to use the physical practice of yoga to support students in opening their hearts, experiencing grace, and letting their inner goodness shine through to the outside world. Classes, which are explicitly sequenced by the instructor or teacher to explore one of Friend's Universal Principles of Alignment, are demanding for both the body and the mind.

Ashtanga

Ashtanga is a once nearly forgotten practice based on the ancient yoga teachings from the Middle East, but it was once again popularized and brought to the West by Pattabhi Jois (pronounced "pah-tah-bee joyce") in the 1970s. It is a more laborious style of yoga that follows a specific sequence of postures and is very similar to Vinyasa yoga, as each style links every movement to a breath. The difference is that Ashtanga always performs the exact same poses in the exact same order, making it a favorite for those who do not always have time to go to a class. Once you have memorized the routine, you are able to complete it wherever you go.

Fair warning: this is a hot, sweaty, physically demanding practice – bring a towel!

Bikram

This type of yoga is the Hollywood favorite! You will see Bikram studios on nearly every corner in some major cities. Approximately 30 years ago, Bikram Choudhury established this school of yoga where classes are held in artificially heated rooms, causing a more strenuous workout. In a Bikram class, you will sweat like you've never sweated before as you work your way through a series of 26 poses. In fact, most classes won't even let you in the door if you do not have a towel (you will need it) and at least a bottle of water. Like the Ashtanga practice, a Bikram class will always follow the same exact sequence, although a Bikram sequence is different from an Ashtanga sequence.

Bikram is also somewhat provocative, as Choudhury has trademarked his sequence and has prosecuted any studios who call themselves Bikram but don't teach the poses exactly the way he says they should or purchase his materials to do the teaching. Since it is so wildly popular, making it one of the easiest types of classes to find and the type that many start out trying. However, it is definitely not for the meek of heart.

Hatha

Hatha yoga is actually a generic term that refers to any type of yoga that teaches physical postures and encourage breathing techniques. Nearly every type of yoga class taught within the West is actually Hatha yoga. When a class is marketed as Hatha, it generally means that you will get a gentle introduction to the most basic yoga postures and principles. You probably won't work up a sweat in a hatha yoga class, but you should end up leaving class feeling longer, looser, and more relaxed. This is a great place to start your practice, as it is a gentle introduction that allows you to see exactly what your body can handle.

Hot Yoga

Hot yoga is basically the same thing as Bikram yoga. Generally, the only distinctive difference between Bikram and hot yoga is that the hot yoga studio deviates from Bikram's sequence in some small way, and so they must call themselves by another name. Some do this for money, others do this because they disagree with a fundamental part of Bikram's philosophy. The room will be heated, and you will still sweat enough to need several bottles of water.

Iyengar

Iyengar yoga was developed and promoted by a mysterious figure identified as B.K.S. Iyengar (pronounced "eye-yen-gar"). Iyengar is a very, very, very meticulous style of yoga, with the utmost attention paid to finding the proper alignment within a pose. This is for those people who are very detail oriented. In order to help each student find that necessary, proper alignment, an Iyengar studio will typically provide a wide array of yoga props: blocks, blankets, straps, chairs, bolsters, and a rope wall are all the most common. There isn't a lot of jumping around, running, or artificial heat, in Iyengar classes so you won't have to get your heart rate up, but you'll be amazed to discover how physically and mentally challenging it is to just stay put. Iyengar teachers must undergo an all-inclusive training – if you have an injury or chronic condition, Iyengar is probably your best choice to ensure you get the knowledgeable instruction you need to not put any unwanted strain on your body.

Restorative

Restorative yoga is one of the best ways for a person who has a lot of stress or is nervous about physical movement in front of others. Restorative classes use bolsters, blankets, and blocks to prop students up in the passive poses so that the body can experience the benefits of a pose without having to exert any unwanted or difficult effort. A good restorative class can be more rejuvenating than a nap. Studios and gyms often offer them on Friday nights, when just about everyone could use a little profound rest. However, they are also available during the week as well.

Vinyasa

Vinyasa (pronounced "vin-yah-sah") is the Sanskrit word for "flow," and that is highly appropriate as vinyasa classes are well known for their fluid and movement-intensive practices. Vinyasa instructors choreograph their classes to smoothly transition from pose to pose, and often play music to keep things lively; however they aren't always the same movements so your body doesn't get too comfortable. The intensity of the practice is similar to Ashtanga, but no two vinyasa classes are the same. If you hate routines or predictability and love to test your physical limits, vinyasa may be the choice for you.

REQUIRED AND RECOMMENDED EQUIPMENT

"A person experiences life as something separated from the rest - a kind of optical delusion of consciousness. Our task must be to free ourselves from this self-imposed prison, and through compassion, to find the reality of Oneness." -Albert Einstein

At its very core, no matter the style that you pick, yoga is about connecting with the mind and body. You can actually practice yoga without any equipment at all if you really wish. Even just sitting and breathing mindfully on a bath towel or pillow as you quiet the mind is a form of yoga that will help you.

However, there are some tools that make it easier, safer, and more effective. Yoga is great in that how much you spend on your equipment doesn't matter as much as what you do with your equipment. When you do a yoga DVD or online video, practice by yourself from memory, or take a class, there are a few items that can help you feel more comfortable. You don't need to go crazy and buy special things that you won't even use, and you really don't need to buy multiples of anything. Here are just a few of the basics that you can purchase to get you through your first few weeks as a yogi. Once you are comfortable, you make your own choices and purchase more or yard sale some of it.

Yoga Mat

If you take a class in a gym, this is probably mandatory. You do not want to use anyone else's yoga mat, as it is probably stinky, sweaty, and full of germs – no matter what the gym says. There are many types of yoga mats, ranging from just a few dollars all the way up to hundreds of dollars. If you plan to practice regularly, invest in a high-quality mat from online or through your gym. Cheaper "sticky" mats tend to fall apart and shed yoga mat confetti all over the place. Consider investing in one that is personalized or stands out, especially if you keep it at the studio, as some people like to do.

Yoga Mat Bag or Carrying Strap

If you're doing yoga at home, you won't need a bag, but if you're going to a gym or a studio, this is a must-have. Without a bag, yoga mats have a tendency to come unrolled at inopportune times, get crushed, or just cause you an inconvenience. Cart yours around in style, and no matter which bag you choose make sure it has at least a small zippered pocket for storing your keys, phone, and wallet! A carrying strap will also help you with storage at home, making it smaller and more compact to slip under your bed or into your closet. Some yoga mats come with carrying straps, so look for the 2-for-1 deals if you can.

Yoga Mat Towel

As stated above, some gyms won't even let you into a class if you don't bring a towel with you – especially if you use public mats. If you plan to practice hot yoga or you just tend to sweat a lot when you're working out, you'll want to have a towel handy to mop the sweat off of your forehead and your mat. Mats, especially cheaper mats, can be slippery and it will prevent you from posing properly. Bigger yoga mat towels typically come with smaller towels to wipe your forehead, and everything matches!

You could use a beach towel, but special yoga-inspired microfiber towels fit perfectly over a yoga mat and are super absorbent. And, these can double as a mat or at least be a barrier between you and that disgusting communal mat at the gym or studio.

Yoga Bolster

Yoga bolsters, also known as yoga pillows, are used to support your body and help you relax in various poses. They are great for beginners, as they can help you stay longer in poses while remaining comfortable. They are also great for older men and women who don't have the strength to hold themselves up. It's a great crux for people who are nervous. You can relax and stretch while you focus on your breath, not supporting your body. These come in different sizes, so it's best to see them in person before your purchase.

Yoga Strap

Yoga straps are an awesome tool for beginners, those who are recovering from injuries, and those who aren't very flexible. They assist during poses where your arms aren't long enough or your body not open enough to reach your feet or other body parts. They also help with stability and give you just a little bit of help when pillows aren't effective. Straps provide length and put limbs within reach. Teachers can also use these as a support to help you go deeper into poses or correct your mistakes. You can use any sturdy rope or scarf, but yoga straps have a buckle to help you create a loop for your hand or foot and won't provide any rubbing or chafing that can hurt.

Yoga Blocks

Yoga blocks are another awesome prop for beginners, the elderly, children, the injured, and yogis of all levels. They can be used as a hand or foot rest when you cannot reach the floor during a certain pose, or they can provide support and stability for limbs or even the back. With their varying heights and a lightweight construction, yoga blocks easily assist with both flexibility and alignment.

POSES FOR BEGINNERS

"You may think that only you are a prisoner, but other people are also prisoners. You are in a small prison, but others are in the big prison outside. When will they be released? Think that you are a yogi and that you are pursuing your sadhana in this particular place and at this particular moment. Immediately you will experience great joy. If you change your understanding, you will be free in a minute." -Baba Muktananda

So you've selected your preferred type of yoga, bought your equipment, and gone to your first few yoga classes and you're a little stuck. Or you're about to go to class and want to be ahead of the curve. Or you really, really want to try yoga, but you don't have the money to sign up at the present time. Well, there are a few different ways to go about learning the basics so that you get the most out of your classes. Study these ten foundation postures, which will be among the very first things you learn as a new beginner, and get a leg up on yoga.

We will describe these poses as best we can, but you might also benefit from going online and looking at these movements in real time. You will want to look at how they get into the poses, move within them, and how they get out of the poses.

1. Downward Facing Dog - Adho Mukha Svanasana

The name of this movement: downward facing dog is almost synonymous with yoga and it's the move that most people picture when they think of yoga. However, just because you've heard of this pose doesn't mean it's easy to do – at least it doesn't mean that it is easy to do correctly. Beginners are often prone to shifting themselves too far forward in this posture, making it more like a plank than the actual movement, putting unnecessary stress on their muscles. So, try to remember to keep your weight mostly on your legs, keep your butt high, and your make sure your heels are reaching toward the floor. Bending your knees a little or a lot is an accepted modification for people with tight hamstrings or those who are not quite in the physical condition to do the movement. Eventually, this pose becomes a resting posture and will be a welcomed relief from some of the other movements.

2. Mountain Pose - Tadasana

Mountain pose may not be quite as famous as the everlasting downward facing dog, but it is every bit as important when you are learning the foundations of all types of yoga. This is a good time to talk about your body's alignment, which is the way that your body parts interact with each other and are ideally arranged in each pose. The alignment in mountain pose draws a straight line from the crown of your head all the way down to your heels, with the shoulders and pelvis stacked along the line on the way down. It is best to think about this as a posture exercise: would you be able to hold a book on your head? A good yoga teacher will talk you through this in class.

3. Warrior I – Virbhadrasana I

This is another one of those famous moves that some people will imitate when they act out yoga for charades. The important thing to remember in the warrior I position is that the hips face forward at all times. Think of your hip points as the headlights on your car. They should be roughly parallel to the front of your mat, and as steady as possible. Sometimes this requires that you move your legs into a wider stance (towards each side of the mat), which will help you feel more comfortable. This movement also requires a little bit of stability and the person that is unaccustomed to the move will waver back and forth for the first few times.

4. Warrior II - Virabhadrasana II

This move is an equally famous slight change from Warrior I. It usually follows Warrior I in sequences. Unlike warrior I, in Warrior II, the hips face the side of the mat, running parallel. When moving as fluidly as possible from Warrior I to Warrior II, the hips and shoulders both open to the side, spreading out laterally. This is a movement that is done a lot, and not just in classes for beginners and it one of the biggest staples. In both warrior poses, aim to get the front thigh parallel to the floor. This will create the burn that will help you burn fat, build muscle and lengthen limbs.

5. Extended Side Angle - Utthita Parvakonasana

This is starting to really amp up your body and push it to the limits. The accepted modification of extended side angle pose is to bring your forearm to your thigh instead of your hand to the floor. This will make it easier for beginners and those who feel aches and pains. The key to this move is for you to stay open across the shoulders. If you reach for the floor too soon or don't hold the pose long enough, it often compromises the position of the torso, making you turn more toward the floor instead of toward the ceiling and making this movement ineffective.

6. Triangle Pose - Utthita Trikonasana

This pose is another one that is deceptively easy looking. It requires quite a deal of balance because your head will start to swim if you aren't focused. It's a great way to practice incorporating your mind into the practice of yoga. Triangle can also cause the same issues as extended side angle, so have a yoga block handy for your bottom hand if you don't think you will be able to do it. You can also rest your hand higher up on your leg, but avoid putting it directly on your knee. Familiarize yourself with the micro bend and apply it here if you want to really push your body to the limits.

7. Cat-Cow Stretch - Chakravakasana

Cat-Cow may be the most important pose you learn when you are just starting out with yoga, especially if you have lower back pain. Even if you never make it to more than a few yoga classes or sessions, continuing to do this stretch on your own will benefit your spinal health and improve your posture significantly. This move requires you to be in an almost crawling position so you might want to put a towel under your knees if you also have some knee pain. Remember that in this position you want to be looking at the ceiling, not the floor.

8. Staff Pose - Dandasana

This one will be a welcomed break for you when you start doing more complicated routines or intensive classes. Staff pose is the seated equivalent of the mountain pose in that it offers the alignment guidelines that you need to know for a host of other seated poses that carry through to all other schools of yoga. You can (and should!) sit on a folded blanket or towel if you have trouble sitting up straight with your butt flat on the floor or you have trouble getting up, as this pose is typically in a movement of other poses. Often this pose leads into a forward bend.

9. Cobbler's Pose - Baddha Konasana

Did you ever do butterfly stretches? Those are similar to this pose. It can also be a good idea to sit up on something like a blanket in cobbler's pose, especially if your knees are way above your hips in this position. Some people even sit with their backs to the wall so they can keep their back in alignment, especially when they are just starting out. Since we rarely sit this way in our everyday lives, especially if we work in an office, this pose stretches some neglected areas of the body. Resort to this pose if you just need a moment of calm.

10. Child's Pose – Balasana

The same can be said about all of the other poses in this book, and many others that aren't even mentioned, but child's pose is really important for you to master. It's the position that you can assume anytime you need a break during a yoga class or during your daily life. If you feel ever feel light-headed or overly fatigued, you don't have to wait for the teacher to call for a break, simply move into child's pose until you are ready to rejoin. No one will say anything, and it is better than giving a half attempt or passing out. It is really up to your discretion, which happens to introduce one of yoga's best lessons: being attuned to the signals that your body is giving you and respecting them above any external directions or inklings you may be getting.

TYPICAL BEGINNING ROUTINES

"Habits allow us to not think about what we're doing . . . giving us the illusion of ease. When we are under the illusion of ease, not thinking about what we're doing. Breathing the same old way, moving the same old way, thinking the same old way we check out of the present, out of happiness itself." -Alex Levin

Here are just a couple lesson plans for yoga classes. This will give you a good idea of what to expect when you go into a yoga class. You can also use them to work at home so that you don't have to spend any money.

Yoga Lesson Plan One

Physical theme: hip-opening poses
Practice principle: patience

Opening (5 minutes)

Begin with Warrior 1. You will return to this yoga pose later when you are done with the movement, as it will show you the difference in your body. If you don't like Warrior 1, you can choose another pose. The pose that you choose should be gentle enough to be practiced without much preparation or warm up. Suggested yoga poses include a standing forward bend with hands on a block for support, reclining pigeon pose (ankle-to-opposite-knee hip stretch) or a reclining one-leg hamstring stretch using a strap.

Only go as far with this pose as you can. You want to be as comfortable as you can be in your chosen pose. Pay attention to the world around you and listen to your heartbeat as you settle into your meditation, if you choose.

Warm-Up (10-15 minutes)

Continue the practice with a dynamic warm-up that will get other muscles moving. This might include cat/cow on all fours, moving between downward facing dog and child's pose or sun salutations. Choose only a few poses and hold them rather than moving through all of them. Feel the movement of the pelvis in these warm-ups, feel it stretch and open up. Think of the muscles as you feel them stretch. Feel how it interacts with your other muscle groups.

Standing Yoga Poses (15-20 minutes)

Choose standing yoga poses that use the hip muscles for strength and steadiness. These poses will create heat within the muscles of the hips and prepare you for more movements. Choose from Chair poses and lunge poses, including the warrior poses if you didn't choose that to start your routine with. Build up to standing balancing poses (such as tree pose) that use the deep rotator muscles of the hips to anchor the balance. During this sequence, focus in on your breathing and feel your muscles straining. Always be aware of your back.

Deep Release (15-20 minutes)

After a sufficiently challenging standing sequence, you will now move to the ground. For this final part of the class, choose a sequence that will stretch muscles all the way around the hip. Seated forward bends, including head to knee pose, can emphasize the hamstrings and lower back. Crossed-legged poses, including cow face pose and spinal twists, provide greater access to the abductors and external rotators of the hip. Seated side bends allow for you to feel how the muscles of the side trunk and low back connect to the pelvis. Low lunges and reclining hero pose open the hip flexors. Bound angle and wide angle forward bend open the groin and adductors. Pigeon pose might be a good apex pose, as it requires openness in many of these areas.

It is during this section that you need to focus in on your breathing and really allow yourself to be at peace and just feel.

Closing (5 minutes)

Go back to the same check-in pose from the opening of your yoga session. How does that pose feel now? Does it hurt less? Can you push your body further? Make sure to make note of the changes that you feel.

Yoga Lesson Plan Two

Physical theme: Twisting from the Core
Practice Principle: Intention

The physical focus of this yoga lesson plan is twisting from the core, and the broader focus of intention mirrors this physical action. You will work to make sure that your core is tight and tones. This is a great abdomen exercise, used by gymnasts. To follow through with our intentions, we draw on our inner strength to support our heart's purpose and direct our actions.

Opening (10 minutes)

You will start your movements with four different core moves that will help align your core and your spine: extension (back bending), flexion (forward bending), lateral flexion (side bending), and rotation (twisting). One possible sequence is to explore extension and flexion on all fours with spine waves (cat/cow), then go into a simple twist. Each movement should be linked to the breath, so make sure you pay attention.

Dynamic Warm-ups (10 min)

You will want to stand during most of this section, as it will cause you to connect with your core and really feel the movements, go through a traditional twisting abdominal exercise (such as the "criss-cross" oblique curl). This is a great time to start doing internal chants if that is part of your typical routine, as you will be doing this movement for quite some time.

Standing Yoga Poses (20 minutes)

You can add a twist to almost any standing pose. Below are some suggestions for adding twists to basic poses. You will want to hold the pose for at least 10 breaths:

- Chair pose (utkatasana) and twisting chair pose (parivritta utkatasana). Have students begin in chair pose, bring their palms together at the heart, twist to one side, and then place one elbow on the outside of the opposite knee.

- Warrior I (Virabhadrasana I) and twisting lunge (parivritta parsvakonasana). From warrior pose, with arms overhead, repeat the transition practiced in chair pose: lower the hands to heart, and twist from the core before placing the elbow on the outside of the front knee.
- Standing head to knee pose (parsvottanasana) and twisting triangle pose (parivritta trikonasana). When moving into the twist from standing head to knee pose, remind students to initiate their movement from the core and not the head and arms.

Make sure you are pushing your body but also respecting the fact that you will need to move the next day!

Seated Yoga Poses and Deep Release (15 minutes)

Choose seated and floor poses that follow the opening sequence of the four movements of the spine. One possible sequence is bridge pose (setu bandh asana) or any other backbends for spinal extension, seated gate pose (parighasana) for lateral flexion, a seated forward bend (such as janu sirsasana) for spinal flexion, and a reclining spinal twist. Breathe.

Relaxation and Closing (5 minutes)

Spend the next five minutes in child's pose, holding the abs tight and reflecting on the class.

CLASSES VS. PRIVATE IN-HOME PRACTICE

"Yoga is the unifying art of transforming dharma into action, be it through inspired thought, properly nurturing our children, a painting, a kindness or an act of peace that forever moves humanity forward."
- Micheline Berry

Once you really get into doing yoga, you will more than likely practice it a few times per day. If you go to the gym every time you want to practice, it is likely to add up to quite a pretty penny. However, there are some distinct benefits to going to the gym. There are also distinct benefits to staying home. It really all depends on how you weigh the pros and cons.

Your pros and cons will be different from the next person's – it all depends on what type of person you are, how much you like to socialize, and how comfortable you are with your body.

What You Will Love About Practicing Yoga at Home

Practicing yoga at home means you won't feel the pressure to compete with anyone else when it comes to your clothing, gear, or poses. You will feel much more relaxed than you ever would in a studio. That is – unless you have kids or pets. Your cat or dog, no matter the type, will sit on your mat or you when you are trying to meditate. It's just a reality.

Yoga at Home

At home, you can go through the movements and poses at your own pace. You can really just focus on yourself, your breathing, and what you are doing and feeling. Because let's be honest, we're all looking at the person next to us in class, comparing ourselves and even copying them. Feeling for yourself and moving your body with the movement, not in competition is the best approach, especially when you are just starting out.

It's also great because you can just put your mat down and start in on your routine. You don't have to wait for others, you don't have to schedule your life around it, and you don't have to wait for the instructor to answer any questions. You have the urge, you have the time, you have the yoga.

Less Money

One of the other biggest benefits is that home practice is free. Some people will think that charging anywhere from $15-$160 for a one-hour class is a little much. There are even some hidden costs: extra if you have to rent a mat, buy a water bottle, buy the shirts they are selling, buy supplements from the person out front, get a box of Girl Scout cookies from the mom who practices next to you, etc. If you do buy a mat or can get a free one, the free ones they usually smell bad especially if you go to a class that's at a gym – always, always, always bring your own mat to a gym yoga class!

At home, you will also be able to put on your own music, wear whatever you want, and go as hard or as soft as you want. Want to practice naked? Go ahead!

So, to sum it up, yoga at home offers:

- Flexibility of your time and efforts
- Complete selfishness in your practice
- Saving cash money
- Controlling your surroundings

What You Will Love about Going to a Yoga Studio

Yoga studios, especially when you are just starting out, is a great place to go because you will be able to start out the right way. Practicing yoga is great if you know how to do the movements. If you don't, it can be a disaster.

You will get adjustments at the gym that you cannot get at home. Even if your significant other is telling you that he or she is helping you – that probably isn't the case.

Some people are uncomfortable with people touching them. If you don't mind being touched, it's a great way to take some classes, perfect the poses, and then drop out and do them at home. You will get the best of both worlds going for that approach.

Going to a class can also help with your stress and emotions. It will completely take you out of your head and you just go wherever the instructor tells you to go. At home, you are surrounded with some of your stressors and are much more likely to think about everything going on around you (like the dirt on the floor that you have to start at while you are in downward dog).

Going to a class at a studio will also help you in learning new ways of going about something, making it harder or push your further. There are so many minor adjustments that can be made in yoga. Although you can try new videos and podcasts regularly, it's not the same as being in a class and having the teacher demonstrate the pose.

In truth, yoga studios are absolutely lovely places. You will be able to socialize with a group of like-minded people who will help push you and make you want to show up for class.

So, to sum it up, yoga at a studio offers:

- Adjustments
- Guided practice
- New ways to do things
- New poses
- Relaxing ambiance
- Socialization

At the end of the day, the choice is up to you. Try out both methods and see which works best for you. Most gyms or studios will offer a few free sessions so that you can see if it is right for you. Don't be afraid to try a few different classes, instructors, types, or studios. This is your money you are spending, it's your body, and it is your decision.

YOGA ETIQUETTE

"You may think that only you are a prisoner, but other people are also prisoners. You are in a small prison, but others are in the big prison outside. When will they be released? Think that you are a yogi and that you are pursuing your sadhana in this particular place and at this particular moment. Immediately you will experience great joy. If you change your understanding, you will be free in a minute." -Baba Muktananda

Yoga-class etiquette is kind of like any other kinds of etiquette: You don't know it exists until you see someone do something seriously wrong. But it is a thing, especially for those who do it regularly. You don't want to be the person who stands out like a sore thumb from the rest of the class. It may take you a while to get acclimated to the feeling of a class, but this is a good starting point.

Chances are, you've committed one of these yoga crimes during class if you've already gone, but not to worry—most people will forget when something happens at the next class. Don't worry about switching classes or moving on to something else. Let bygones be bygones.

However, if you haven't started yet, jot down this list and remember some of the universal hard and fast rules for yoga classes:

1. Don't stroll into the room 15 minutes late with Starbucks, like a college senior who just doesn't feel like going. No one likes that person in college, and people really don't like that person when they've been in camel pose for two minutes and have sweat running down their faces. Show up at least ten minutes early and be respectful. If you are going to be late, sit out that class and wait for another one.

2. Don't hog the prime spot in the room. You probably have your favorite spot in the classroom—by a breezy window that allows you to have some air, by the water cooler, underneath the skylight, in front of the instructor, right near the door for a quick exit—but be flexible. A Saturday morning yoga class can get pretty packed, and you don't want to be that guy who refuses to move his mat three inches to the left because it'll ruin his view.

3. Don't bring your iPad, iPhone, iPod, i-ANYTHING into the room. This is a calm space and people don't need to hear your Nicki Minaj ringtone in the middle of child's pose. This also goes hand in hand with another rule that's for the gym, in general, not just yoga: do not post selfies during your class. You are supposed to be working out, and whoever is behind you does NOT want to be flattered in that way.

4. Don't walk across other people's mats to find a spot to roll yours out. Someone's face will be centimeters away from that or even touching it. Can you imagine the germs that are on your feet? Or even worse – your shoes? Just don't do it.

5. Don't under dress. You might think that because it is so hot that you can wear a tiny top and short shorts. However, the people in your class do not want to see anything happen during class. You are not Janet Jackson and the rest of the people in your class are not your gynecologist or proctologist.

6. Don't wear the same yoga pants for an entire week straight. Yoga pants are cute and sometimes they can be quite expensive. But just because you're going to ruin your clothes with sweat again the next day, that doesn't mean you should throw personal hygiene out the window. The person next to you will appreciate the fact that your clothes are freshly laundered and you don't smell like an Italian hoagie or worse. The same goes for your mat: make sure you sanitize or air it out every once in a while. No one likes a cheesy mat.

7. Don't talk to the person next to you about how your ex cheated on you with someone he met on OkCupid or how your sister had to get sewn up after she had her baby. Chances are, you are oversharing and no one cares. Instead of focusing on telling the entire room about your day, focus internally on calming everything down. If you have so much to say that you can't stop yourself from talking, you need to focus more internally than ever.

8. Don't laugh at yourself, your friend that slipped and fell, or the 80-year old man wearing an Abercrombie Speedo in the front row. You will hurt feelings and you might stop people from ever coming back. Things will happen: people will slip, someone will do a move wrong, someone might fart, or someone will look incredibly dumb. Chances are, it can happen to you as well.

9. Don't be a sweat hog and not clean up after yourself. Practicing yoga, especially hot yoga or Bikram, can get you pretty sweaty, so bring a towel. Dripping sweat all over your neighbor's mat is a bit like peeing on a stranger's carpet, it isn't recommended. If you know you sweat a lot, try not to use the community mats. You might also want to invest in some towels or absorbent clothing.

10. Don't Stare.

11. Don't Stare.

12. Don't rush out of class like the building is on fire. Everyone else wants to get out of there too – wait your turn and be polite.

Following these simple rules of etiquette will certainly make your time as well as everyone else's time at the studio a productive and enjoyable one.

CONCLUSION

"Yoga, an ancient but perfect science, deals with the evolution of humanity. This evolution includes all aspects of one's being, from bodily health to self-realization. Yoga means union - the union of body with consciousness and consciousness with the soul. Yoga cultivates the ways of maintaining a balanced attitude in day to day life and endows skill in the performance of one's actions." -B.K.S. Iyengar

In the end, yoga is more than just sanskrit and poses.

The purpose of Yoga is to create harmony in the physical, vital, mental, psychological and spiritual aspects of the human being. You might be doing it for some exercise or to improve one aspect of yourself, but in reality it is working on all of them at the same time.

In the previous pages of this book, you have learned quite a bit about the practice of yoga, what the use, where to go, what to pick, and how to do it. The rest of your journey with yoga is deeply personal and up to you.

Yoga is not mere practice for an hour or two in a day a few days a week, but it is the most scientific way of living, all the twenty-four hours of the day. You will be transformed by yoga if you give it the chance to help you grow and change as a person.

Convert your life to the ways of yoga, so that you may ensure success in all the fields of activity of your professional life to your romantic life. By regular practice, by using your presence of mind, skill and wisdom, you can become Yogis and enjoy happiness and peace, whatever be the circumstances and conditions in which you are placed.

How much yoga changes you is up to you.

Namaste.

Sid Akula

Don't forget your FREE Bonuses at:
www.plaid-enterprises.com/yoga

www.ingramcontent.com/pod-product-compliance
Lightning Source LLC
Chambersburg PA
CBHW070524290526
45790CB00003B/1289